Midwifing Death

In loving memory

of my brother

Angelo ('Tony') Barbato

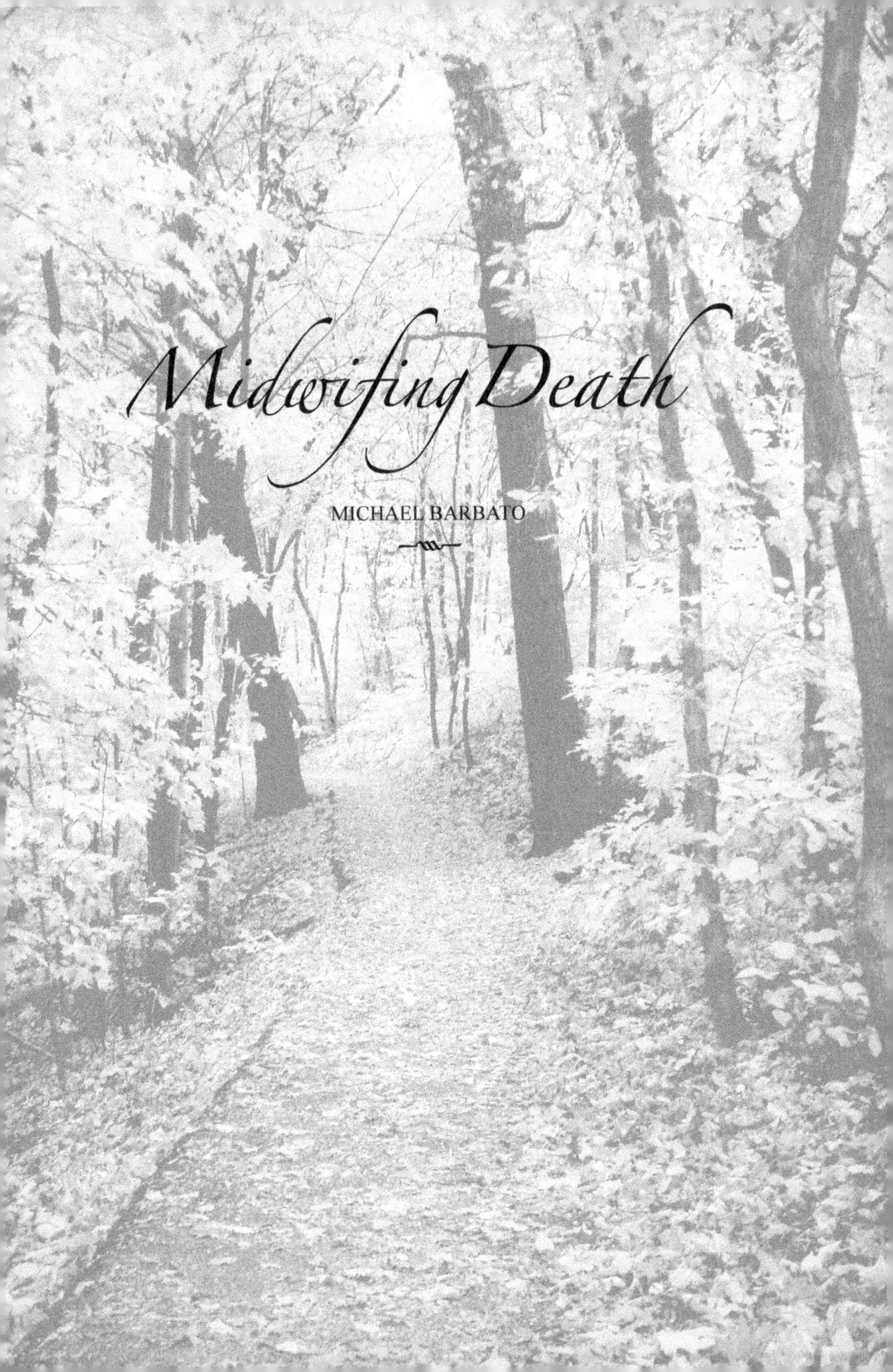

Midwifing Death

MICHAEL BARBATO

National Library of Australia Cataloguing-in-Publication entry:

Barbato, Michael
Midwifing Death

1st edition 2013
Reprinted 2014, 2015
Includes bibliography

ISBN 978 0 646 59555 9

Subjects: Terminally ill
Terminal care
Holistic nursing
Death – Psychological aspects

Dewey Number: 362.175

Cover and interior design: Ruth Barbato

Printed on 70GSM classic by Griffin Press, Adelaide

Other publications by Michael Barbato:

Caring for the Dying (2002)

Reflections of a Setting Sun (2009)

Caring for the Living and the Dying (2010)

www.caringforthedying.com.au

Acknowledgements

I acknowledge and thank my patients and their families for the valuable lessons they imparted as they lived the experiences I attempt to describe throughout this book.

As with the last two books, *Midwifing Death* is a family affair. I wish to thank Ann, Claire, Ruth, James and David for their encouragement and for the faith they have shown in me. A special thanks to Ann and Claire who proof read the final manuscript and to Ruth for applying her exceptional graphic design talents to the cover and internal layout.

I gratefully acknowledge permission to reproduce the following copyright material.

The cover photo 'Forest Path' with permission from Sherri Dunham of Budding Lotus Transformations.

Quotations from the book *Magnanimous Despair* by Grahame Jones, copyright 1998, reprinted with permission from Boombana Publications, Queensland.

A quotation from the book *The Spectrum of Consciousness* by Ken Wilber, copyright 1993, reprinted with permission from Theosophical Publishing House, USA.

A quotation from The Wings of Night (*Holistic Nursing Practice*) by Janet Muff, copyright 1996, reprinted with permission from Wolters Kluwer Health, USA.

Passages from Symbolic Expressions of Dying Patients (*Nursing Forum*) by Daniel Dugan, copyright 1989, reprinted with permission from John Wiley and Sons, USA.

Quotations from the book *A Place of Healing* by Michael Kearney, copyright 2000, reprinted with permission from the author.

A quotation from the book *Pluto's Republic* by Sir Peter Medewar, copyright 1984, reprinted with permission from Oxford University Press.

Quotations from the book *The Art of Being a Healing Presence* by James Miller, copyright 2001, reprinted with permission from the author James E Miller and Willowgreen Publishing, Indiana.

A passage from the book *Men's Business, Women's Business* by Hannah Rachel Bell, copyright 1998 and published by Inner Traditions International, Vermont.

Requests for permission to quote from the following sources have gone unanswered or are pending.

Quotations from the book *A Death of One's Own* by Gerda Lerner, copyright 1978 and published by Simon and Schuster, New York.

A quotation from the book *The Hour of Our Death* by Philippe Ariès, copyright 1981 and published by Penguin Books, Middlesex.

A quotation from the book *The Road to Daybreak* by Henri Nouwen, copyright 1988 and published by Doubleday, New York.

A quotation from the book *Facing Death* by Robert Kavanaugh, copyright 1974 and published by Penguin Books, Baltimore.

A passage from the book *Kitchen Table Wisdom* by Rachel Naomi Remen, copyright 1996 and published by Pan Mcmillan, Sydney.

A passage from the book *The Enlightened Mind* by S Mitchell, copyright 1991 and published by Harper Collins, New York.

Contents

Introduction

Introduction

It is a little more than twelve months since my older brother was diagnosed with acute myeloblastic leukaemia. Until then, Tony had been extremely fit and healthy. In his youth he was a champion athlete and footballer, having played in a Sydney-based Rugby League competition alongside the legendary Reg Gasnier. In later life he swam, walked and cycled, played competition golf, maintained a large garden and attended to his many bonsais. His only health problems were the legacy of his many sporting injuries. He was, in fact, recovering from surgery to a torn muscle in his shoulder – the consequence of too much golf – when a routine blood count requested by his general practitioner revealed the tell-tale signs of leukaemia. Even before the doctor broke the news Tony sensed something was amiss; he gripped the waiting-room chair and anxiously awaited his fate. Her demeanour was unmistakable; he anticipated bad news, but not leukaemia. That word felled him like some vicious blow. He knew he had been delivered a death sentence and his previously safe world shattered in an instant.

Although stunned, he managed to walk home where he shared the devastating news with his partner and immediate family. Disbelief and dread filled the air. There was, however, little time to ponder the implications of this newly made diagnosis as Tony found himself in a hospital bed within two hours of leaving the doctor's surgery. In a matter of days he was transferred to a larger hospital 350 kilometres from home where momentous decisions had to be made. The nature of the disease was explained, and the pros and cons of chemotherapy were laid bare. There was no hope for cure but treatment, he was told, could induce a brief remission adding one or possibly two years to the otherwise grim prognosis of three months. Tony weighed up his options and with a minimum of fuss he chose not to proceed with potentially life-prolonging medication. This courageous call was made because a decision in favour of treatment would have entailed several months away from home. The thought of being separated at this time from those he loved was intolerable. He considered that to be a fate worse than death.

Despite dire predictions Tony wanted to maintain his precious normality. His way of living and the relationships that enriched his life were now more important than ever. He wanted to share whatever time he had left with his partner, his three children, grandchildren, siblings and close friends. He chose to live out his remaining days at home rather than languish in hospital. The wish to preserve his cherished way of life was more important than the possibility of a few extra months, a large part of which would be spent in hospital enduring the burden and side effects of chemotherapy.

After a few good weeks Tony's blood count deteriorated and his brief sojourn at home was threatened when doctors advised urgent treatment within the local hospital. This sudden, but not unexpected setback brought back the spectre of imminent death and weakened Tony's earlier resolve to forego all active treatment. Reluctantly, he submitted to the doctors' recommendation and packed his bag for hospital. On arrival he received blood and platelet transfusions, and while these reduced the risk of haemorrhage and the need for oxygen, his morale suffered greatly. Tony wanted to live, but not as a patient. He did not want to die, but he did not want to live this way – dependent on treatment that offered no hope of cure, while at the same time compromising his independence and way of life. His experience was similar to that described by Grahame Jones in the book *Magnanimous Despair*,

> *"What I detest is how effectively the procedures rob me of my precious normality and seriously affect my morale. The dehumanising rites of [treatment] plunge me into an abyss of discouragement that I could never describe... humanity goes and one becomes a something, a clinical something, attached to the laboratory equipment"* (1998: 35-36).

Tony's spirits may have hit rock-bottom, but it was this very hospital experience that gave him the courage to say, enough is enough. After five days he asked to be discharged and freed from the never-ending rounds of investigations, interrogations and interventions. To their credit, the doctors reluctantly bowed to Tony's wish even though they expressed concern about the challenges that lay ahead, and how the family would cope. Tony's life was hanging by a mere thread. His family, although daunted by the task confronting them, chose not to shirk the challenge or the responsibility. They did not want his death to be hidden behind hospital walls as if it was too frightening to witness or too difficult to manage at home. They wanted to honour Tony's wish to return home and to die in his bed, and for them to minister to him until the very end.

But, who would guide the family along this crucial, but unfamiliar journey? They needed someone who could liaise with the doctors and nurses, enlighten them about death's ways, sustain and support them in their caring endeavours, advocate for them, and open them to the mystery of death and the extraordinary gifts that are on offer, even in the face of such immense sadness. What they needed was someone who could midwife the dying process – *an amicus mortis* (a friend of the dying) – who, according to Ivan Illich, is not afraid of the bitter truth and is willing to stay to the inexorable end (1995: 3).

Death is not simply the end of life – defined medically as the absence of a pulse, a heartbeat and respirations. It is a profound human experience. The threat to one's very existence is a much more painful burden to shoulder than the travails of the physical body. For this reason those confronting death need more than a skilled technician. They need someone who is prepared to venture into uncharted waters. Someone who can be present to the dying person as they silently plumb the depths and hidden passages of their soul. Apart from pastoral care workers, chaplains and volunteers it is rare to find someone within or outside the hospital environment who is willing or capable of fulfilling this role. In her book, *A Death of One's Own*, Gerda Lerner writes about the death of her husband and her indebtedness to an amicus who taught her how to meet death and accept it. She says,

> *"To have such a person at such a time is a great good fortune. To be that person, to have been such a person is a*

> *heavy and blessed experience. Once in each lifetime, we are meant to be a blessing [an amicus] to another"* (1978: 133).

Sadly, medical successes have come at a cost. The importance of midwifing death has been steadily eroded within the hospital environment, and technology has all but replaced the human touch. More time is now spent interfacing with computers and writing reports than at the bedside in meaningful dialogue with patients and their families.

Fortunately Tony had his midwife (several in fact) who guided, supported and advocated for him and his family. Between them, they did everything possible to ensure Tony's physical, emotional and spiritual needs were met. His final weeks were spent at home with the ones he loved, sharing cherished stories and saying painful goodbyes. His health, however, deteriorated rapidly and following a brief period of unconsciousness he finally submitted to death's embrace. It was a surreal moment for all the family who had gathered beside him. There was enormous sadness, but also relief and gratitude that his wish to die at home had been met.

Caring for a dying loved one
takes you to the ultimate threshold
of transformation and renewal.

John O'Donohue
Anam Cara

This book looks at the role of an amicus in midwifing the death of another, and presents a model of care that attends to the whole person. This model is not only appropriate for those whose death is predictably close; it can also be used for anyone living with a life-limiting illness, even if their life expectancy is measured in months or years. The practice of midwifing death focusses on an individual's response to the threat of death and the need for them to preserve their dignity, their autonomy and their much cherished *precious normality*. One day you may be called upon to be an amicus for a relative or friend. This book prepares you for this most important humanitarian role.

Chapter 1

The changing face of dying

Chapter 1

The changing face of dying

I graduated at a time when the medical care of dying patients left a lot to be desired. In that pre-palliative care era, dying patients were discreetly moved to an area of the ward where they were least visible, and the curtains discretely drawn around them (there were few single rooms in public hospitals back then). While this was done ostensibly for the benefit of other patients, it poignantly symbolised the denial some doctors harboured concerning death. Dying patients under the care of these doctors were sometimes hurriedly dealt with on ward rounds in the belief there was nothing more that could be done. Philippe Ariès described this human tragedy as the *Invisible Death* – where silence and indifference not only denied patients the truth but also the opportunity of saying goodbye. This was not only a denial of death, it also disregarded its significance.

While this reflects poorly on the medical profession as a whole, the doctors themselves were not callous; they mistakenly assumed their work was complete when cure was no longer possible. This attitude was reinforced by two entrenched beliefs – that a doctor's objectivity could be blinded if he/she became overly concerned with their patients' circumstances, and that truth-telling did more harm than good. Many in the medical profession considered silence to be the best course of action here. In many instances they also convinced the family to maintain a charade of hope in the presence of their dying loved one. Collusion on such a scale did not, however, hide the truth, it simply made the journey lonelier and more painful for the patient and family. The consequence of such actions was described by Ariès as follows,

> *"The last inspiration of this inventive affectivity was to protect the dying from his own emotions by concealing the seriousness of his condition until the end. When the dying man discovered the pious game, he lent himself to it so as not to disappoint the other's solicitude. The dying man's relations with those around him were now determined by a respect for this loving lie"* (1981: 612).

As a junior doctor I was often caught up in this 'loving lie' and would find reasons not to visit dying patients unless called. I would go out of my way to avoid their relatives, but if cornered I found myself reassuring the family that everything was being done, rather than raise the real issue of impending death. I had great difficulty in admitting the truth. There were many reasons for this, and while my memory for these times has glazed over, I believe my discomfort stemmed from a fear of how people would react to the 'D' word. The fact is, I was the one who was uncomfortable with death and conveniently convinced myself that truth telling in these circumstances created unnecessary suffering and was best avoided. Without realising, I had put my fear of death before the needs of my patients and their family.

Whole-person care

Thankfully, the medical profession has realised the error of its ways, and care of the dying has slowly improved. This is largely due to the pioneering work of the late Dame Cicely Saunders who saw a need for the medical profession to alter its attitude towards death as well as its approach to care. She believed more could be done to ease the suffering experienced by dying patients, and in the mid-1960s she introduced a philosophy of care that is now known throughout the world as palliative care. She maintained that those whose illness was beyond cure needed *whole-person* care. This not only meant appropriate pain relief and comfort measures but also the opportunity for them to dialogue with significant others or, as Cicely Saunders would say, to share that which occupied their heart as well as their mind. She believed the dying needed a good communicator as well as a competent doctor. Someone who would not only ensure their physical comfort but would also hear their suffering and that of their family. Someone who could facilitate the openness and honesty that circumstances such as these require. Death is not something we can skirt around. It is a profound human experience worthy of our time, our care, our respect and our reverence.

Palliative or whole-person care is not radical or new. Its roots go back centuries, to medieval times when places of rest existed to provide food and shelter for sick and weary travellers. Over time, these places became hospices for the dying. They were predominantly staffed by nuns who considered their institutions to be "stopping places for the soul on its journey to God" (Lewis 2007: 20). While there was little in the way of medical services, the dying were lovingly cared for in an environment where death was held in awe.

In this largely secular world, the earlier hospice orientation towards the hereafter has now been replaced by a model of care that is still person-centred, but more outcomes orientated. Pain relief, comfort measures, autonomy, dignity and attention to suffering have supplanted salvation as the ultimate goals of care.

While these goals have become the cornerstone of contemporary palliative care, the sense of mystery surrounding death has not been lost nor has the humane touch that respectfully honours the uniqueness of each individual been forgotten.

Despite this shift towards whole-person care, dying, according to Alan Kellehear has become a "shameful affair" because of the mistaken sense of failure that is perceived to accompany it (2007: 8). This is rarely the case when death occurs within an aged care facility or a palliative care unit, but is more likely to be true when efforts to prolong life have been intense or protracted. Death in this clinical environment is often accompanied by the pain of unfulfilled hopes, irrespective of how forlorn they may have been. If dying is not given the respect it deserves, death is accompanied by the pain of loss and also a gaping wound of disbelief. In the case of sudden and unexpected death this wound festers as family relive the last moments and confront the inevitable and endless 'if onlys' and 'what ifs'.

The first death I witnessed was that of my grandmother some 65 years ago. She had cancer of the stomach. No treatment was available and she, like so many others at that time, died at home. There was much sadness and crying, but there was no sense of failure. In today's era she, almost certainly, would have been hospitalised, subjected to numerous tests and offered chemotherapy and/or surgery. Her family's hopes would have been buoyed with the seemingly endless options available, and one can understand the disappointment they would have felt when told that all the treatments had failed. Death under those circumstances can only result in a sense of defeat, and her family, like so many others today may have "raged, raged against the dying of the light" (Thomas 1939). In so doing, they would have been blinded to her gentle passing and would have grieved her loss even more.

The medicalization of death does not prepare us for what lies ahead. It is as if we hold our breath, close our eyes, and fail to see or hear what we instinctively know to be true – that death is approaching. It is times like this when we need someone who can midwife the dying process and open our eyes to reality. This time-honoured art has been an unintended victim of medicine's success and was, for several generations, all but forgotten. It has, however, found a new home for expression in palliative care, and the opportunity for family to journey with their dying loved one is once again possible.

Midwifing death

The art of midwifing death has been practiced for as long as humans have lived (those seeking more information on death through the ages are referred to Ariès 1981; Kellehear 2000 and 2007). Not so long ago, the definition of a good death was one where the person's eternal salvation was assured. The emphasis therefore was on the state of the dying person's soul rather than their physical comfort. For centuries, it was the priest who attended the dying, and it was he who midwifed the dying process. In the early-mid 15th century, when the population of Europe was decimated by the Black Death, few priests were available or willing to attend the masses of people who were dying – an estimated 20 million people or one third of the population then living in Europe were thought to have died in the space of two years. Given their role, it comes as no surprise to know the number of clergy that died was proportionally higher than that of the general community. More than 50 per cent of their number perished, but a significant number also abandoned their post fearing they too would suffer the same fate. With this number of deaths, and with few clergy who could or would attend, manuals were developed to guide families as they ministered to their loved ones. This was the beginning of the *ars moriendi* tradition, or of family and community midwifing death.

The possibility of laity midwifing the death of family or friends became possible with the publication, in the mid-15th century, of what is now known as the *ars moriendi* (The Art of Dying). This manuscript was so highly regarded that by the end of the 15th century it was available in all the major language groups throughout England and Europe. The *ars moriendi* is in fact an abridged manuscript of the much longer *Tractus Artis Bene Moriendi* or *Speculum Artis Bene Moriendi*. These texts are composed of six sections and include a series of prayers, quotes from Christian authors, instructions on how to die, a list of five temptations that might arise and compromise the dying person's salvation, and instructions for how family could assist the dying during their final hours (Campbell 1995).

The *ars moriendi* is comprised of the five temptations alone. Unlike the *Tractus* it also includes inspirations that were used to overcome the corresponding temptation. Each temptation together with its equivalent inspiration occupies one page and a related image is located on the opposite page. These ten pages form the bulk of the text, suggesting that it was designed to be a simple and practical guide for the masses, many of whom were illiterate.

The *ars moriendi* tradition of midwifing death continued for centuries, but lost favour as people became more secular and moved away from Catholicism – the religion to which the text was originally orientated (Leget 2007). Its death knell came with the advent of modern medicine, which brought with it the hope of cure. The dying no longer gave in to what was previously considered inevitable, and the pursuit of survival has now become the dominant theme. Death moved from homes to hospitals, and a family of willing carers has been replaced by a well-drilled healthcare system.

The sequestration of death to places outside the home has not only seen the *well-managed death* (Kellehear 2007) replace a natural death but has also led to a form of disempowerment that renders most families helpless and vulnerable in the face of death.

In recent years, many in the community have become disillusioned with the nature of care given to the dying, and medicine itself now sees a need to 'do death better'. Once again families seek to be more involved, but there is little to guide them in the way of caring for their dying loved one. The time for reviving the lost art of midwifing death has arrived – not to replace the science of care, but to instil within it the art of caring.

The use of the word *midwife* in relation to death may seem unusual; even paradoxical. In the context of birthing we understand a midwife to be a nurse who is present for, guides and assists an expectant mother as she moves through the various stages of labour. The person who midwifes death has exactly the same role, only the context is diametrically opposed. In the past it was always a member of the clergy or, in their absence, a relative or friend who midwifed death. Today it could be one or more family members, a palliative care volunteer or a pastoral care worker. In recent times the term *amici mortis* (friends of the dying) or *death doula* have been used to designate those who take on the role of midwifing death (Illich; Grogono; Elliot). Their work is both challenging and rewarding, and any willing adult, working in unison with a general practitioner and palliative care team, is capable and worthy of this role. Indeed, there is something hauntingly beautiful and awe inspiring about midwifing a relative or friend through this major life transition that we call death.

The late Dr Elisabeth Kübler-Ross often told the following story. As a universally aclaimed authority on death and dying, Elisabeth expected hospital patients would seek her out as their death neared. Much to her chagrin it was not her they asked for, but the woman who served tea within the ward. Elisabeth was puzzled and asked this woman, "Why do they ask for you and not me; I'm the expert?" In reply, the woman simply stated, "Death is an old friend." As it turned out she had been an amicus to many of her own family and was familiar with death and its mysterious ways. She was not afraid to sit with those in the ward who were dying, and to be present to their needs. Her presence was more than a comfort; it was a source of strength that the dying person and family could draw upon. It was as if her presence was the means by which sadness, grief, fear, anxiety, anticipation, love and reverence could melt into one incredible experience. The very presence of someone who is not afraid of death is the blessing or amicus that Gerda Lerner was so thankful for.

Where people die

The majority of people in Australia if given a choice would prefer to die at home, yet fewer than 20 percent do so. Most die in hospital, a palliative care unit or an aged care facility. Fear of the unknown, the responsibility of caring for someone who is dying, paralysing grief, and a fear of falling at the last hurdle can be so overwhelming a dying person is often transferred from their place of residence to a hospital or hospice at the eleventh hour. The nature of the illness or accident, its suddenness and severity can also be factors in determining the place of care. Similarly, extenuating family circumstances, social factors, carer exhaustion and the lack of community services may play a part. In some cases the transfer is prompted by the hope that something more can be done to prolong life. It may also come at the recommendation of others, including the attending medical practitioner.

Transfer to a hospital, hospice or aged care facility frees the family from much of the hands-on care and decision making. Despite this, fear and the not knowing remain, and are no less paralysing for these families as they are for those who midwife death at home. The fear is now compounded by an unfamiliar clinical environment where all one can do is wait, watch and hope. To their credit, these facilities have recognised the anguish family members endure and now utilise pastoral care services to inform, support and sustain a family throughout their ordeal. In a 2012 ABC Compass documentary, pastoral care workers were described by grieving families as a blessing or a gift. They brought a much needed human touch to a medical scene, which is as foreign as it is frightening. Some families referred to them as 'angels'. I prefer to call them *amici*.

In most (but not all) circumstances, there is much that could be done to support the family and to facilitate a person's wish to die at home. The provision of improved community services probably tops the list, but close behind is the need for an amicus to midwife the dying process – to guide, inform, support and advocate for the dying person and his/her family. The physical and emotional demands in caring for a loved one at home are challenging, but my experience tells me they are not insurmountable. If families are given the necessary support, most would willingly take on this onerous, yet rewarding task. All we need are more people who are prepared assume an amicus role.

Our Indigenous cousins show us how death can be midwifed despite the countless challenges. Regardless of distance and level of services, they do all they can to ensure that another of their 'mob' dies in his or her own 'country'. The very thought of dying in hospital is abhorrent to them, and contrary to their long-established beliefs and customs. It is not unusual for an Aboriginal person to be transported hundreds of kilometres so they can die at home. Family members choose to midwife the death in a way that is unique to their culture and country, and they do this with limited resources and facilities.

HOME is where the soul or spirit resides; the space which holds the most cherished memories and gives meaning to a person's life. This may be a place of residence, a particular location or something beyond the ordinary. When a dying person says, as they often do, "I want to go home", they are often referring to a place of peace that can only be found beyond mortal existence. For them, "I want to go home" suggests they are ready to let go of life.

Today's amicus

The crucial attributes of an amicus include a genuine compassion for those in need and an innate capacity to love. If you can come to terms with your fear of death and equip yourself with information, you have all that is needed to fulfil this role. This book will help you to address these two important elements. It introduces you to the art of midwifing death and to a healing model of care. It gives you information on the basic needs of the dying person and introduces you to a way of being present to yours and your loved one's needs.

Experience tells me that those confronting death desperately need a companion, preferably a family member or friend, they can trust. Someone they can open up to if and when the need arises, who does not offer advice or false comfort, and who can hear their deepest cry without feeling they must make things better. Someone who can sit comfortably through silence and stillness, and 'hears' what is *not* being said without resorting to irrelevant or endless questions. In essence, this companion is fully present to whatever the moment brings.

Knowledge alone will not prepare us for this task. We can only make this journey if we are prepared to look deep inside and confront our own fears around death and dying. One day you may want to be an amicus for someone you love. Whether that person's death occurs within the home, hospital, hospice or aged care facility, this book is a first step in preparing you for the role of midwifing the death of another.

The next chapter will open with an exploration of what is meant by 'healing in the face of death'. It will then introduce a practical model for midwifing death – a contemporary *ars moriendi*. While healing is always the desirable outcome, it should never become the prime agenda. Indeed, it has been said that any agenda to heal will always get in the way of healing. Generally speaking, people die the way they have lived and any process that fails to respect this can do more harm than good. The only goal for those who midwife death is to be present for the person dying. Midwifing death is more about *being* and less about *doing*.

Chapter 2

Healing in the face of death

Chapter 2

Healing in the face of death

Healing is a term commonly employed these days to describe the gradual resolution of grief that follows the death of a loved one or a tragic event that grips the mind of many. The process of healing may be personal and private, but could also be part of a ritualised public outpouring as seen with the death of Princess Dianna and following the recent Sydney siege. The process of coming to terms with tragedies that do not involve us directly is relatively rapid. We grieve for the pain and loss of others, but quickly return to our previous state of being and way of life. The story is different when the tragedy involves us intimately as with the death of a loved one. Then, the healing process is more profound and protracted.

What is hard to conceive, however, is how healing can occur with those who are dying? It may come as a surprise, but healing is more likely to occur at life's end than any other time in one's life. For those who are left to grieve, the death of a loved one is painful beyond measure, and for the one who is dying the experience is as surreal as it is frightening. There is, then, a desperate yearning for both the carer and the cared-for to communicate at a level that goes beyond the normal sharing and conversation of everyday life. They may want to express their love and appreciation for each another, speak of joyful times or seek forgiveness for events, often minor and long past, that caused or continue to cause pain. The outcome of such heart-felt exchanges may be a coming together as never before, bringing with it a sense of profound peace. In the words of one author, a person may be blinded by tears, but enlightened at the same time (Livingstone 2000).

The paradox of something painful resulting in something good is represented archetypically in the image of the snake. Michael Kearney, a palliative care physician writes, "The serpent has always stood for two diametrically opposed ideas, namely the foe of mankind on the one hand, and as man's protector and saviour in disease and distress on the other" (Kearney 2000: 59). Like the snake, healing in the face of death is something of a contradiction, but only if we make the error of equating healing with cure. Healing does not signify recovery from illness. It means 'becoming whole' or, in the words of Michael Kearney, "becoming more completely who we are" (2000: 60). I prefer to think of it as rediscovering rather than becoming – a return to a state that once was rather than a journey towards something new. The words of Michelangelo may clarify this distinction. When asked how he created such beautiful sculptures from blocks of marble, he replied, "The beauty is always there; all I do is remove the excesses."

When given the opportunity, those who are dying will seek to shed their excesses – the emotional baggage they, like all of us, accumulate throughout life – and in the process they rediscover some or all of the peace they once knew.

"This gift of time to prepare for death has had
a powerful effect on me...I like the person I am becoming
more than I have liked myself before."

DR J BARTHOLOME

Healing is a blend of many possibilities, most notably peace, love, acceptance, forgiveness and self-forgiveness. While the outcome is much sought-after, the journey towards healing is rarely smooth. Opening to fear and other emotions can be as painful as it is cathartic. Occasionally the emotional pain may be so overwhelming that people remain captive to it, incapable of freeing themselves from that which causes their suffering. Dying may be tough, but to die with all one's pain locked inside can lead to despair and intolerable suffering. Such a death is anything but peaceful and may be a source of anguish for the one dying and for those who are left to grieve. Sadly, this is a relatively common scenario, and may say more about a lack of time and the low priority given to preparation for death than it does about the individuals themselves.

One of the criticisms of modern medicine is the lack of opportunity given to the sick and dying to express their fears and their anguish. There is a busyness that surrounds illness. A busyness confined almost exclusively to waging war against that which causes ill health, distracting the attention of the care team from the all important business of seeing how the person and not just the patient is faring. There is no reason why healthcare cannot be personalised and given as high a priority as any other dimension of care. All it takes is a shift in attitude – where *being* is seen as important as *doing*.

When death is inevitable, it is more humane if desperate attempts to prolong life give way to truth-telling. The sick have an instinctive feel for when death is near, and know when the truth is being withheld. Deceit only adds to their pain and isolation (read Leo Tolstoy's *The Death of Ivan Ilyich* to better appreciate the suffering that accompanies collusion and deceit). The bitter truth may hurt, but I am often told the not knowing is harder to bear. For any number of reasons – usually fear of upsetting the dying person – doctors, nurses, family and friends may be reluctant to deliver bad news. The dying person senses this and suffers in silence and their journey towards healing is severely compromised.

> *Recently, I heard the story of a 90-year-old woman who was dying at home. On the initial home visit, the palliative care doctor was met at the front door by one of the daughters who said, "Don't tell mum she is dying. She is old and frail and will not cope with the news." The doctor questioned her about this, but the daughter was insistent that her mother not be told the truth. The doctor then entered the mother's room while the daughter waited in another part of the house. After the usual pleasantries the mother said to the doctor, "Please don't tell my daughter I am dying, she will not cope with the news."*

Healing presence

There is a well-known adage that people die the way they have lived. Although this is occasionally true, I believe all who are dying, irrespective of their past or present behaviour crave peace. The reason it may be hard to come by often stems from a lack of opportunity or a lack of courage – attempts to prolong life may assume greater importance or the dying person may be reluctant to talk about their pain. Most commonly, it is because nobody is prepared to listen.

Healing is not about making people feel better. Nothing can be 'done' to take away the pain of dying, but an environment can be created which may facilitate the healing process. Healing can only come from within. It cannot be dispensed or passed from one person to another. It is a process of self-transformation that may arise unexpectedly, but more often follows the opportunity to unburden oneself – to let go of troubling thoughts and emotions while another person listens and hears the pain that is being expressed. The other's role in this exchange is to 'simply' listen and be present to the dying person's immediate needs. This role is far from passive nor is it easy. It takes someone, "Who can be silent in a moment of despair or confusion, who can stay with bereavement, who can tolerate not-knowing, not-curing, not-healing and face the reality of our powerlessness" (Nouwen 1988).

This healing presence could be a relative, a friend, or a member of the medical or nursing profession. Occasionally it is a total or relative stranger. The characteristic they share is that the person is prepared to listen without giving advice (something that is unfamiliar to most). Listening helps create the environment where the healing process can begin. Where the other not only speaks of their pain but also experiences it as though reliving it. Sharing in this manner is a way of letting go of whatever is causing suffering. It is the essential first step towards healing and is heavily dependent on having someone listen – a healing presence.

I cannot know myself except
through the intermediary of another person

J. P. Satre

The prospect of being the one who hears another's pain may be daunting. To be chosen, however, is a validation of how you are esteemed by the other. It is the gift the dying person offers you, and your *presence* is nothing short of a blessing in return. It not only indicates your willingness to accompany the other as they enter the labour phase of dying but also shows that you are prepared to enter into their pain.

A holistic model of care

In her book *Men's Business, Women's Business*, Hannah Rachel Bell, describes how the Ngarinyin people of Western Australia enter into and share the experience of childbirth as they midwife a birth,

> *"When her time comes, the women take her [the expectant mother] to their special place for birthing...they prepare a fire, collect water, special leaves and herbs, and sing... the women attend the birth assisting its process with song,*

> *rubbing, chanting, warmth, medicines and reassurance. The father is taken to special place some distance away where older men loosen all his restrictive clothing and tie a hair belt around his girth. He lies back with his legs wide open and pulls on the belt ends to assist his wife to give birth to the child with his energy... he transmits his energy and breath to his wife"* (1998: 38-39).

This example illustrates how we can be fully present to another's suffering when we share in it. In Western cultures, fathers can now enter the delivery suite and share the experience, if not the pain of childbirth. While this is a long way removed from the way of the Ngarinyin people, it does at least give men in Western societies an insight into labour, and allows them to better empathise with their partner's pain and the experience of birthing. The same applies to death. We can only empathise with another's pain and suffering if we are fully present to them and their experience, share their vulnerability and relinquish control of the moment.

This book presents a holistic model of palliative care that will help you prepare for the labour of love involved in midwifing the death of another. The model transcends the narrow view of health and sees illness as something that affects the whole person. The notion of the body as a machine, of illness as the machine breaking down, and of the doctor as repairing the machine is an outdated and dehumanising model of care (Engel 1977). Illness affects the whole person, their body, their mind and their spirit. When death is inevitable, it is the death of the *person* we know and love that makes dying such a profound experience, and why a model of care that acknowledges and attends to this is so necessary. That is not to say there is no place for a model that attends to the machine. Medicine has a very important role, particularly in pain relief and the palliation of other troublesome symptoms. There is, "A large and profoundly important scientific element in medicine, there is also an *indefinable artistry*, an *imaginative insight*, and medicine is born of a marriage between the two" (Medawar 2002). This is particularly true when caring for someone who is dying.

Now, more than ever is the time to ensure this marriage is consummated and becomes an accepted model of care for all those living with a life-limiting illness. There is a need for a modern-day *ars moriendi*. A model of care that meets the needs of the secular, culturally diverse, and ageing society we now live in, while at the same time respecting each individual's desire for autonomy, self-determination and a pain-free death (Leget 2007). The following illustration introduces readers to a healing model of care and the four key domains to midwifing death. Each of the four domains are equally important, and while they will be considered separately, it should be remembered they are part of a package that constitutes whole-person or holistic care. The next chapter will concentrate on the science of care and the provision of physical comfort while subsequent chapters will focus on the 'indefinable artistry'.

> *Many people wonder where they should be and what they should do, when in fact they should be more concerned about how to be.*
>
> MEISTER ECKHART

The four domains to Midwifing death

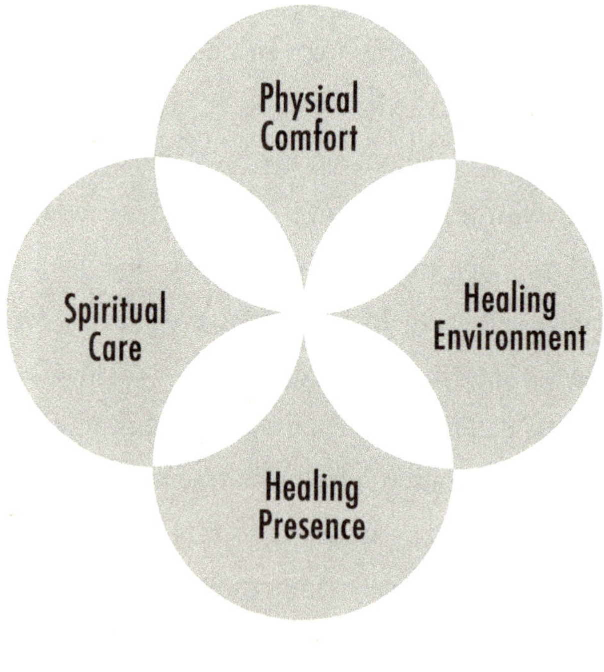

Chapter 3

Physical comfort

Chapter 3

Physical comfort

We all carry within us the seed of death. Woody Allen's terse comment, "No one gets out of this world alive" is a haunting reminder of the destiny that awaits us all. Despite its inevitability, very few give death a second thought unless they themselves are confronted by it, or when a family member or close friend dies. Try as we may, the thought of not existing is hard to comprehend. It is as incomprehensible as it is unspeakable. Fear accounts for why so few acknowledge death's reality and prepare for it. Epicurus first spoke of this some two thousand years ago when he said, "A person fears death not because it will be painful, but because it is painful in anticipation". Psychologists consider the fear of death the greatest of all fears; too frightening for us to contemplate.

For those burdened by a life-threatening illness, the fear of death is, however, real and ever present. As their illness progresses and treatment options become fewer and more burdensome, the frightening reality of impending death dawns. Most ultimately resign themselves, albeit reluctantly, to their inevitable fate and what they come to fear is not death, but what they may have to endure beforehand. This fear is often compounded by the memory of having seen others, usually parents or grand-parents die in pain or struggling to breathe. Although this memory may be many years old, the bearer of such a memory invariably anticipates a similar fate.

The reassuring assertions of palliative care cannot eliminate such painful memories, but palliative care can change the way people die. There is now a broad range of treatments for most symptoms encountered towards the end of life and the dying no longer suffer the way our predecessors did. Intractable or interminable pain is a thing of the past. The palliation of distressing symptoms is eminently achievable and is an important goal of palliative care. Physical comfort, however, only marks the beginning and not the end of whole-person care. Distressing symptoms not only result in unnecessary suffering but also limit a person's ability to engage with the ones they love; to enjoy what remains of their life and, ultimately to prepare for their death. Only when comfort is achieved can those who are confronting death open up to what really matters.

Doctor Richard Lamerton acknowledges the clear link between physical comfort and whole-person care when he says, "Palliative care *firstly* seeks to make a person's body a comfortable enough place to live in so that he or she can, if they so choose, prepare for death" (Lamerton 1980).

Palliation of symptoms

Palliative care has dramatically improved the quality of life for people living with a life-limiting illness. The most remarkable change has been in the relief of painful and disabling symptoms such as pain, breathlessness, nausea and vomiting which, in the past, frequently undermined a person's will to live as well as their way of life. The goal of achieving physical comfort is, as Richard Lamerton suggests, given top priority in palliative care. Details of treatment, including the names of medications used are not detailed here, but are available in my earlier book, *Caring for the Living and the Dying.*

What needs to be stressed is that relief of symptoms is achievable. If symptoms do not improve when medication is first prescribed, doctors will incrementally increase the dose until the desired effect is attained. If this fails or side effects intervene a change in medication may become necessary. Sometimes it takes days or longer for the desired goal to be realised. This is no reflection on a doctor's competence. It is simply a matter of finding the right dose of the right drug. If the situation is more pressing, doctors may recommend admission to a nearby hospice or hospital where the process of determining the best treatment can be safely accelerated.

Overall comfort

Physical comfort does not depend on drugs alone. Comfort involves more than the absence of pain and may be compromised or improved by all manner of things. One of the most common concerns, particularly amongst those who are frail and confined to bed, is bodily discomfort. It often hurts to be touched, moved or turned. Even lying in bed can be uncomfortable. Detailed attention to the bed, the mattress, the weight of the coverings and the way the person is nursed can make the world of difference. If the person is nauseous or has lost their appetite, the sight or smell of food can add to their distress. Excessive noise, constantly ringing phones, slamming doors, unnecessary interruptions, the ambient temperature and the level of lighting all influence the way a person feels. There is no need to go into detail, but it is important to appreciate that what troubles them may not trouble you, and vice versa. This is particularly true of food and, to a lesser extent, fluids. Irrespective of the underlying illness, those approaching death lose their appetite, and their reduced intake often becomes an unnecessary focus of attention. In the absence of other causes, loss of appetite and a reduced food intake is to be expected. In the face of death, love rather than food is far more sustaining.

If there is a problem, approach it with compassion and understanding. If you are unsure, or if the measures you or others institute fail to resolve the difficulty, seek help from others. Assistance is always available and is as far away as the phone.

The role of an amicus

While the choice of treatment for the palliation of symptoms is left to the professionals, an amicus has the important role of ensuring the dying person's pains are adequately heard and addressed. This is particularly true when care is situated within the home. In one of the very few articles that appear in the medical literature on this topic, Dr James Grogono, a consultant surgeon who midwifed his wife's death at home, stresses the importance of what he calls shared care (2000). The palliative care team may recommend treatment, but it is the family in their role of amicus who alerts the palliative care team of a problem, administers the prescribed medication and monitors progress. They carry a heavy burden of responsibility and are therefore an important part of the palliative care team. They need to be informed about all aspects of treatment; dosage, frequency of administration, the potential benefits and side effects, and how to respond if treatment fails to achieve the desired goal. This information together with an action plan in case of worsening symptoms or unexpected complications is best documented in writing. As things have a habit of going wrong at the most inopportune time, after-hour contact details (preferably mobile phone numbers) for the general practitioner and the palliative care team should also be available. Remember, the task of an amicus is not to manage symptoms, but to ensure medication is taken as prescribed. In the event of worsening symptoms they should contact the prescriber and advocate for the one they care for.

Knowledge is power, and amici are in a better position to advocate for their ailing relative or friend if they are well informed about their loved one's symptoms and their current medications. This is true irrespective of the place of care – home, hospital, hospice or aged care facility. Myths and misinformation particularly in relation to pain-relieving medication will be dispelled and side-effects of treatment will be recognised earlier. Apart from reporting symptoms or new developments, amici can also advocate on behalf of their loved one on any number of issues, particularly when that person is unconscious or incapable of making their wishes known because of dementia.

Those without a healthcare background may think the advocacy role is beyond them. My experience tells me otherwise. An amicus, because of their relationship to the one they are caring for, is better positioned to midwife that person's death. They know the person and not just the patient, and will therefore have a better understanding of their needs and wants as well as their state of mind. Doctors and nurses have the skills to effectively manage a dying person's symptoms, but they lack the strong personal connection of an amicus. The palliative care personnel and family make an excellent team, capable of delivering whole-person care.

Advocating for a dying loved one is integral to the role of an amicus. An amicus is ideally placed to ensure preferences for how a person wishes to be cared for are carried out. Hopefully, this has been discussed well in advance, agreed upon and documented in an Advance Care Directive (ACD). The need for advance care planning and the subsequent documentation of a person's preferences cannot be stressed too highly. The conversations required to achieve this may be difficult, but they can have a profound healing effect on the carer, the immediate family and the one being cared for. On a more pragmatic level, an ACD removes the onus of responsibility from family for the difficult end-of-life decisions that may have to be made. The role of an amicus is to ensure the wishes of their dying loved one, as documented in the ACD are honoured, thereby facilitating a most important goal of care – allowing that person to *die their own death*.

Death as a release

Although the fear of death is said to be universal there are some who, for any number of reasons, welcome death and see it as a release from their suffering. The despair they feel is not that they are dying, but that they are still alive. They are ready and more than willing to embrace death, either because life has been too long or because it is too hard. Their journey is also painful, and the need for an amicus is equal to that of any person facing death. If they are to *die their own death* they too need someone they can trust; someone who can hear their unusual brand of pain.

The experience of imminent death

The late Elisabeth Kübler-Ross once said, "Dying is like taking off a tight shoe." This may or may not be true for the one who is dying, but for those left to grieve the path towards death is rarely seen in such a positive light. Gerda Lerner's experience of watching her husband die is probably a truer reflection of how most perceive the death of someone they love,

> *"[A] level of misery, growing almost imperceptibly greater each day, but seemingly bearable because it sways slightly – somewhat better here, somewhat worse there...all told, each day is ever so slightly diminished...the silken cord*

> *[of death] begins to draw the net closer again – tighter, tighter"* (1978: 182-3).

Later in the book she says,

> *"How do you chart the incoming tide, the rhythmic pattern of wave upon wave, the slight increases in peaks and troughs, the imperceptible advance of tide's edge?"* (1978: 199).

Some days, the prospect of death may be viewed by the patient and family as a blessed release; other days it is much too close for comfort. This is the experience of living between two worlds – the world of the living and the world of the dying, of the known and the unknown, the world of hope and that of fear. Grahame Jones highlights the dying person's struggle when he says, "I still feel full of life, the desire to live, but I am tied to a body whose very existence has been undermined on all fronts" (1998: 105). Another of my patients expressed similar sentiments when she said, "I do not want to die, but I don't want to live this way." It goes without saying the experience of living between two worlds is also true for family and friends with one important difference; they witness, but do not experience death.

As I sat with my brother during his final hours, when he was unconscious and could no longer communicate, I wondered what it was like for him. Was he suffering or was he beyond suffering? I believe, and there is some evidence to suggest, that at this stage of a person's life they are in a deep sleep and more peaceful than most of us would consider possible. My palliative care experience told me that Tony was no longer in pain, but I also knew the family's pain would shortly reach new heights.

How you can be present during these final hours is something I will take up in later chapters. But for now, permit me to share my thoughts about what may transpire at this time. I will begin with the dying words of a young woman I cared for several years ago. Almost imperceptibly she was heard to utter the following, "I feel as if I have left my body." Although she died immediately after this revelation, I have no doubt of what she was telling us. She was not only free of her body but she was also free of the struggle to breathe that had plagued her during the latter weeks of her illness. Peace came in the last moments of her life because she was, only then, free of that tight shoe – her disease-ridden body. This woman had an out-of-body experience (OBE) at the moment of her death.

Out-of-body experiences most commonly occur as part of the near-death experience (NDE). Near-death experiences are frequently described by those whose life is threatened by serious illness, a motor vehicle accident, drowning, a fall from a great height, et cetera. Very early in the incident, the person's consciousness suddenly 'leaves' their body and the disembodied self witnesses everything from a nearby position. They feel none of the pain associated with the illness/accident, but can see what is happening to the body they have left behind. There is no fear or anxiety only peace, and enormous love and compassion for the body they once occupied. This phenomenon is a common accompaniment of the NDE, and was first described by Raymond Moody in *Life after Life*.

Those who are dying have similar near-to-death experiences, and these are called deathbed visions (DBV). As the name suggests DBVs commonly occur at the moment of death, but may also manifest days or weeks before. They are frequently accompanied by a vision of a pre-deceased relative. On occasions the vision is so vivid and seemingly real it wakes the person from their moribund state (Wills-Brandon 2000; Fenwick & Fenwick 2008). To witness such an event, as I have, is remarkable and leads one to wonder about the significance of DBVs as well as their cause. A DBV is, in almost all cases, a joyful and comforting experience for the one who is dying and does, in its own mysterious way, fast track the healing process. The powerful healing quality of a DBV is revealed in a recent anecdotal report in which a series of DBVs not only prepared an elderly woman for death but also her family (Estle 2013). More information on OBEs, NDEs, and DBVs can be found in my earlier book, *Reflections of a Setting Sun.*

A feature of the OBE, NDE and DBV is that the mind not only dissociates from the body but it also seems to 'change channels' – it moves from fear to a place of peace, freeing itself from the pain and mental anguish that may have been present beforehand. Lesser degrees of dissociation also occur with deep sleep, meditation, contemplative prayer and day-dreaming. Even though the person's mind is in another world, these forms of dissociation are different to an out-of-body or deathbed experience per se. I prefer to call them *out-of-mind experiences* (OME). The person is no longer in their troubled discursive mind, but has transitioned into a more peaceful state. Michael Kearney, a respected palliative care physician well-known for his interest in *soul pain*, suggests these 'deep mind states' are doorways to the unconscious which, "Contain, often in the most unlikely and darkest corners and in the most unexpected of disguises, exactly what is needed to deal with the particular question, challenge or life crisis that confront us" (1996: 56).

While in this state, a person is not only free of the mental torment that characterises their wakened state but are also in a timeless space where nature can instigate healing. The better the sleep, meditation, et cetera the greater the dissociation and the resulting peace. In the context of dying, these states should not be regarded simply as periods of rest, but as times of potential healing. Paraphrasing the words of the poet Robert Frost, these states can make all the difference.

Out-of-mind experiences are more likely to occur and are more powerful when a dying person is pain free. While there is no proof, there is every reason to believe these altered states of consciousness may contribute more to a dying person's improved quality of life and state of mind than hitherto realised. For this reason, everything should be done to ensure times of sleep, meditation, and even musing are respected and safeguarded. Relief of pain and other troublesome symptoms help to achieve the optimal conditions, but peace and quiet are also necessary. Sudden or loud noises are particularly disruptive and disturbing. We are all familiar with the disorientation that occurs when we are woken suddenly. Everything, therefore, should be done to ensure these times, even brief daytime naps, are not disrupted. This is one of the many tasks of an amicus.

All that has been said about OMEs apply equally to the time of unconsciousness or coma that often precedes death. Unconsciousness can be likened to a deep sleep and should be afforded the same respect as sleep. Provided the person receives appropriate pain relief, this period is also a time of healing. More will be said about this fascinating world of the unconscious or deep mind in Chapter 7. Before doing so, however, we will turn our attention to the second of the four healing domains – the environment that surrounds and envelops the sick and dying.

Chapter 4

A healing environment

Chapter 4

A healing environment

When asked to speak to community groups about palliative care I often start by asking one simple question, "Where would you like to die, at home or in hospital?" The result of this straw poll is invariably the same – most prefer to die in their own home. This does not surprise me, but I often wonder why, in this highly medicalised society, people prefer a home death to one within a hospital where professional help and support is readily available? The answer probably lies with the all-important succor and sanctuary found in the familiar routines of a 'homely' environment; luxuries that are sacrificed within a clinical setting. Next to comfort, those at the end of their life value relationships and connections more than anything else. They desperately seek to maintain what Grahame Jones calls *precious normality*, much of which is lost in the course of an illness and is ultimately extinguished with hospitalization.

Precious normality

Humans, like many in the animal kingdom experience grief, but are unique in that they alone anticipate loss and prepare for it. In the face of the slowly encroaching and ever consuming penumbra of grief, it is little wonder the dying seek to preserve as much of what they hold dear – their precious normality. The company and intimacy of those they love invariably tops the 'precious' list. A distant second, but nonetheless important, are visits by family and friends, all manner of conversations, home comforts, routines, a favourite chair, a favourite room, and freedom to do as one chooses; all of which are severely compromised when someone enters hospital. Hospitalisation and institutional care not only robs the sick of things that are integral to their life, they also lose a large part of their identity.

Tony grieved the loss of his precious normality during his times in hospital. It made those stays intolerable. The excellent care could not make up for what had been lost. His precious normality was more life-sustaining than the blood transfusions and other treatment available to him in hospital. We are creatures of habit and the people, routines and connections that make up our precious normality become *vitally* important when death threatens. One of the important tasks of an amicus is to assist their sick or dying loved one retain as much of their precious normality as possible. This takes some creative thinking if your loved one is dying other than in their home. The more medicalised the care, the harder this is to achieve.

Several years ago I was part of a team caring for a seventeen-year old girl dying of cancer. She had been hospitalised because of severe pain and while this gradually came under control her remorse increased as it became increasingly clear she would spend her eighteenth birthday in hospital. The family made plans to celebrate the occasion, but what made this young girl's day was the effort of the ward doctor who filled her room with colourful balloons while she was being showered. On her return she was overcome and shed tears of joy. This little show of thoughtfullness altered her mood and changed her day.

Precious normality and dementia

If any assurance is needed about the importance of precious normality, one only has to consider the example of people with dementia. Within this group, things that were once precious or normal cannot be recalled, but are not forgotten. Although beyond the reach of words, things that are precious remain deeply embedded in that person's psyche (Sherman 1999). People with dementia may not remember names or recognise faces, but powerful sensory clues such as a memorable photo, a much-loved item of clothing, a favourite perfume or a familiar tune, will often bring tears of recognition. Given this, any attempt to change long established patterns of behaviour can have consequences.

Barbara Sherman, in her book *Dementia with Dignity* gives the example of a woman who caused a disturbance every time her carers attempted to shower her in the evening. When they learnt that she always showered in the morning, the familiar pattern was re-established and the 'problem' was promptly solved (1999: 77). Recently, I was told of a woman who had made several valiant, but unsuccessful attempts to abscond from a low-level care unit. Fortunately she was always found at the nearest bus stop. The staff made some inquiries and discovered she had, in previous years, caught the bus to work. The nursing home built a mock bus shelter within the grounds and would regularly take the resident to sit there. No longer did she attempt to escape. There are also instances of people with dementia who continue long-established habits such as jogging and gardening even when they can no longer hold a conversation.

Long term memory and precious normality are deeply imprinted and better preserved in those with dementia than is short term memory. Re-establishing links to these memories may make a difference to the life of the person living with dementia. While words are meaningless, renewing these once important connections may be the key to midwifing the life and death of a person with dementia.

It has been said that the Alzheimer journey is a kind of passage from the mind into the heart. People with Alzheimer's may not remember, but the emotional connections are basically intact. For this reason 'speaking' to their emotions is a more powerful avenue of communication than language. They may have lost their short-term memory, but long-term memory and intuition is preserved well into their illness. Never underestimate the ability of people with dementia to recall their emotional links to the past. Those interested in this subject are referred to Barbara Sherman's excellent book (see bibliography).

Creating a healing environment

When Tony left hospital for the last time I took leave from work and assisted the family in midwifing his death. I was not sure what awaited me or how I could best help. I need not have worried for Tony had very quickly eased back into his familiar routine. He woke at the same hour each morning, had his usual breakfast of cereal and toast and then took a leisurely stroll around the garden.

A routine of daily chores followed, but these were now completed by family under his watchful eye. Morning tea was taken as he had done for many years before, always in his favourite chair, and within sight and smell of his beloved garden. Lunch was followed by an afternoon nap, visitors, and a final stroll around the garden before dinner. He completed the day sitting with family watching the evening news before retiring to bed. Although some of these activities were taxing, he maintained this routine until the very end. This was clearly important to him, and in many ways this regular and ordered life sustained him during those final weeks.

Creating a healing environment is not difficult when caring for someone at home. It is really a question of maintaining as many of the familiar routines as is possible, and trying not to let the delivery of care overtake the *caring*. There will, of course come a time when the need for medical care surpasses all else, but even then the healing environment can be maintained by the loving manner in which the care is delivered.

The task is a little more testing if your loved one is in a hospital, hospice or an aged care facility. Creating a healing environment outside of the home involves good communication, a little imagination, and a modicum of organisation. It is a little more challenging, but not impossible. The closer you are to the person, the more certain you can be of what they might want. Aim to stimulate all the senses – sight, sound, smell, taste and touch – remembering the sense of smell has the strongest connection to memory and is most likely to evoke a response even in those who are seemingly unresponsive. Loving actions and unexpected surprises, no matter how small, can be profoundly rewarding. I know of a family who recorded steam train whistles to play to their father as he was dying in hospital. This man had been a steam train driver for much of his earlier life. This action proved to be as healing for the family as it possibly was for the man himself.

Hearing and the sense of touch are present until the very late stages of life. Playing a person's favourite music, reading to them, reciting a well-known prayer, talking to them, holding their hand or brushing their hair can be enormously comforting, even when they are unconscious and close to death. To hear they are loved and how they have enriched the life of others is perhaps the greatest gift we can offer at this stage of their life. To be held, kissed and nurtured in this way often gives the dying person the strength to ultimately let go of life. I will say more about the ability of unconscious patients to appreciate sound and touch in Chapter 7.

Chapter 5

A healing presence

Chapter 5

A healing presence

While preservation of precious normality and attention to the environment are essential to midwifing death, the most important space you prepare is, according to grief counsellor and Protestant minister, James Miller, "Not around you but within you" (2001: 30). Based on his own personal experience, the psychologist, Robert Kavanaugh draws attention to the negative influence fear may have on human interactions. He says "... most important, I found that those around me who were not busy running from their fears could be my closest and only effective friends as death came near" (1974: 57). The harmful effect of running from fear is best illustrated in the following report,

> *Lou, a 54-year old man with metastatic brain cancer, told his nurse, "Last night, suddenly, the nurses came and got me and flew me all the way to China. They put me all alone, on one side of the Great Wall. I knew my family was there, on the other side of the wall, but I couldn't see or hear them, or reach them in any way. It was terrifying. Please don't let them do that to me again." The nurse walked over, took Lou's hand, and said firmly, "Now, Lou, we didn't do any such thing. You were here in the hospital all night sleeping like a baby."*
>
> *During the previous week, Lou had spoken at length of his feelings of isolation from his family. His wife and two teen-aged daughters visited him regularly each evening for brief periods, after they had finished their work and school activities. Despite his obvious and dramatically deteriorating condition, his wife repeatedly assured Lou during her visits, "We need you at home, you know, so hurry up and feel better so you can get out of here." Lou expressed feelings of isolation and frustration in the face of his family's denial of his dying and their own emotional pain* (Dugan 1989: 24).

Lou's wife, blinded by grief as well as fear, could not face the reality of her husband's impending death. The 'loving lie' she chose to live may have been a deliberate, but futile attempt to protect Lou from the truth. She was unable to sense Lou's need for closeness, honesty and intimacy, and the emotional dissonance only served to separate them further from each other. Sadly, she could not be the healing presence that Lou desperately needed (it is important to note that the nurse also failed to hear Lou's pain. She sought to placate rather than hear his cry for help.)

Contrast Lou's story with that described by Rachel Naomi Remen in her book, *Kitchen Table Wisdom*. Here, the art of being a healing presence seems so simple and uncomplicated.

> *"At first she had driven her mother to her doctor's appointments, shopped for food, and run errands. As her mother grew weaker, she had prepared tempting meals and cleaned the house. When her mother stopped eating, she had listened to her and read to her for hours. When her mother slipped into a coma, she changed her sheets, bathed her and rubbed her back with lotion...In the end she just held her and sang"* (1996: 45).

Elisabeth Kübler-Ross often told the story of a mother of two young children who was dying of cancer. She asked this woman to speak to a small gathering of people about the sense of isolation she experienced throughout the course of her illness. The woman started her talk with a simple question, "How would you feel if you were visiting me in hospital?" Some said they would be anxious about what they should say, others were frightened about saying the wrong thing, others were angry that a young mother was dying, while others expressed concern for her children. "You see," said the woman, "therein lies my problem; you are all so concerned about something, none of you is sufficiently empty to hear my pain."

Ideally, family, carers and visitors should leave their emotional baggage 'at the door'. A preoccupation with one's own agendas may impair the capacity to be present to the needs of another. It is difficult to hear or sense suffering if the focus is on what we should or shouldn't say or what we should or shouldn't do. This 'background noise' reduces our ability to hear and to be fully present, and is a diversion from the real task at hand.

There is no faking it here. Those who are dying are extremely intuitive. They can see through any pretence and will respond accordingly. Emptying yourself of all distracting thoughts and emotions allows them to engage you in a manner of their choosing. They may chat, hold meaningful dialogue or remain silent. Your open demeanor is a gift to the dying – it gives them permission to be as they choose at that moment.

Recent studies have shown that the human brain contains 'mirror neurons', so called because they are activated by the mere act of observing – actions performed by one person activate the exact same pathways in an observer's brain. If, for example you watch a game of tennis, your mirror neurons will be activated in the same way as if you were playing (Rizzolatti, Fogassi & Gallese 2006). Imagining playing tennis will do the exact same thing. This explains why visualisation is thought to enhance performance and why it is recommended by many sporting coaches.

The relevance of this to midwifing death is that people who are highly intuitive (the dying *par excellence*) can sense what another is experiencing *viscerally*, and they then experience the same emotion. They not only perceive another's fear but also their compassion and equanimity. Caring for self, a commitment to reflective practices and awareness of underlying agendas go a long way to ensuring that an amicus is a healing presence for the one whose death they are midwifing. We can only be present for others if we are, first and foremost, present to ourselves.

When death is imminent, the dying almost always seek to have their immediate family close by. The loving presence of someone they know and trust is a source of comfort, and this sustains them throughout their final weeks. It offers opportunities for both to reminisce, engage in meaningful dialogue or simply share the stillness. Love, honesty and authenticity are what make this connection meaningful. There are, of course, other essential tasks which increase in number and complexity as a person's illness progresses, and while these are mandatory, the importance of being fully present to the other's psycho-spiritual needs should never be compromised because of the doing. So, what does it take to be a healing presence?

A healing presence is someone who is aware and responsive to what is happening at that moment. He/she is equally aware of what motivates them – their fears and agendas – and ensures, as best they can, that these inner forces do not compromise their capacity to hear what is said or what remains unsaid. The message is clear – we can only be present for others when we empty ourselves of our own fears and needs. It is this that ultimately determines the quality of another's presence. In the words of James Miller, however, "Being present is simple, but that doesn't mean it's easy" (2001: 14).

People who possess the qualities of a healing presence do not resort to quick fixes or look for ways to make things better. They do not use words to soothe a troubled mind, fill silences with questions and comments, or engage in futile activities. These manoeuvers may deceive the carer into believing they are responding appropriately, but they do not deceive the dying person. Despite their physical state, those close to death are aware of agendas that motivate others. They are highly attuned to body language and pay more attention to this than to any words or actions. They understand *viscerally* what is in the mind of another.

True listening brings us in touch even
with that which is unsaid and unsayable.

JOHN O'DONOHUE
ANAM CARA

Communication and patience

There are no words which adequately convey the feeling of what it is like to die; the experience is ineffable and incomprehensible. John O'Donohue says, "When you are lost in the black valley of pain, words grow frail and dumb." For this reason, questions like, 'how are you?' or 'how do you feel?' while well-meaning are often met with silence, a look of apprehension or a glib "I'm okay." "The mind falters" says Gerda Lerner, "It draws a dark curtain and refuses to function" (1978: 200). So, how do you communicate with a relative/friend you know to be dying?

In his book, *I Don't Know What to Say*, Robert Buckman suggests there may be times when nothing needs to be said, and that silence and body language are more powerful than the spoken word. Body language carries more weight than words, and has a wonderful innate intelligence. John O'Donohue emphasises the dangers when we pre-empt a situation and plan our words. He says, "Your mind can deceive you and put all kinds of barriers between you and your nature; but your body never lies." Our body speaks to us; it alerts us to our agendas and our fears and directs us to act from the heart rather than be misled by the mind. Authenticity should underpin all our efforts to communicate. The reward for such integrity is that quality of presence will always speak louder than words. More than once I have said something that I regretted only to be told subsequently that my presence and compassion mattered more.

Some of the most unnerving times for anyone engaged in conversation are times of silence. Silence is often perceived as an unintended pause, a vacuum or empty space waiting to be filled – for life to be breathed back into the conversation. Silence is none of these; it is an opportunity in waiting and an exercise in patience. The usual mistake is to assume that nothing of worth takes place during these times of silence when indeed the opposite is true. Phil Barker, a Professor of Psychiatric Nursing Practice says, "People who wish to learn the art of caring need to begin with the exercise of patience" (2000: 100). Rainer Maria Rilke describes how this is done,

> *"Being an artist means: not numbering and counting,*
> *but ripening like a tree, which doesn't force its sap, and*
> *stands confidently in the storms of spring, not afraid that*
> *afterward summer may not come. It does come. But it*
> *comes only to those who are patient, who are there as if*

eternity lay before them, so unconcernedly silent and vast. I learn it every day of my life, learn it with pain I am grateful for: patience is everything" (Mitchell 1991: 186-187).

Patience is the ultimate test of a person's mettle and their capacity to be a healing presence. It is also what dying patients look for in us. They value the highly skilled and competent carer, but when the chips are down they want a healing presence – someone who can cry with them as well as laugh, who is sensitive as well as practical, is open to what each moment brings, and does all of this without trying.

Metaphor

As I sit with those who are close to death, I am amazed by the powerfully evocative language they manage to unearth. A retired medical practitioner, dying of breast cancer said to me, "I am climbing a tall mountain and when I get to the top I have to do an appendix operation. I am frightened because I have not done one before." When the family heard this, they believed she was hallucinating because of the morphine. I knew from experience, however, that she was using metaphor to tell us that death was nigh, and she wondered what she needed to do to die well. Once her words had been decoded and their meaning understood, the family's initial concerns were eased and they were able to comfort, support and be present for their mother throughout the final phase of her journey.

When words fail, we not uncommonly resort to metaphor. This is particularly true for those who are dying. Their experience is indescribable, and the only way they can adequately express themselves is through silence or metaphor. All too often the significance of the metaphor is lost within a hospital environment, and the words are often misconstrued and attributed to an hallucination resulting from morphine, other medication or illness. My concern is that family and friends believe the medical interpretation and are distressed by the thought their loved one is dying in a state of confusion. What could be a gift (albeit in disguise) is, unfortunately 'lost in translation'. Hallucinations certainly occur around the time of death, and sometimes they may be medication-induced, but like a dream these seemingly confused ramblings often hold the key to something profound. When Greg, a man in his early twenties with widespread cancer said to his parents, "I want to go home" everyone thought he must be hallucinating. Greg died a few hours later.

Metaphor may be used to gently alert family to a truth they do not want to hear or cannot accept. Greg's family would not accept the fact he was dying and his words, "I want to go home" were lost to them and also the medical team. On another occasion, an elderly woman said to her daughter, "I wish I could fly away like that yellow bird." The daughter had cared for her mother over many years and was troubled by the thought that she might die on her watch. Indeed, she did everything in her power to ensure her mother's continuing survival. The mother's message was clear; she was ready to let go – to take off the tight shoe that Kübler-Ross spoke of – but before she could do this she wanted her daughter to know that death was a welcome relief from the suffering she had endured throughout the years. In saying this she released her daughter from any guilt she may have felt over her inevitable death. This was the mother's final gift to her daughter; a gift the daughter ultimately accepted.

There is now mounting evidence to suggest that those who are dying are likely to resort to symbolic language when attempting to convey an important message. This is often the only avenue available to them, as ordinary language fails with something as incomprehensible as dying. But, because the message is frequently obtuse there is a danger the words will be attributed to the effects of the illness and/or its treatment. This was the case when a patient who was close to death announced to her family that she was going on a beautiful holiday (Barbato 2010: 138). We need to take careful note of what is being said, and not jump to conclusions. If you don't understand, seek clarification by asking the person to tell you more. Silence and holding the person's hand are equally good responses particularly if the person has withdrawn into him/herself. In situations such as these, the dying person's body language may be more helpful than their words. If they are calm and introspective, be patient and don't assume the obvious.

Truth telling

Those who are dying are highly intuitive and can sense when someone is uncomfortable or when they are withholding the truth. Not uncommonly, I am asked to refrain from giving bad news, particularly if it's to be directed to an elderly or young family member. There may be genuine reasons for such a request, but more often than not it is made in the mistaken belief that 'bad news' will only add to the other person's suffering. Truth telling may be painful, but if done with sensitivity and compassion it engenders a level of trust that can only strengthen the bond between the people concerned. Truth telling does not eliminate suffering, but it gives everyone the opportunity to come to terms with reality and to focus on the things that are important. Neither of these is possible when truth is withheld. Everyone suffers when we perpetrate or perpetuate a '*loving lie*'.

The motivation behind the loving lie is a genuine desire to not add to the suffering of someone who is dying. As worthy as this may sound, withholding the truth or offering false hope simply delays the inevitable and denies the person an opportunity for healing. The truth ultimately makes itself known and the resulting disappointment and/or confirmation of what they suspected all along but were never told causes more pain, for now it is accompanied by a tragic loss of trust. Truth telling is painful, but deceit hurts more.

Several years ago a middle-aged man of Mediterranean descent was admitted to our palliative care unit following surgery and radiotherapy for a malignant brain tumour. His family informed me that he was not to be told of his diagnosis as it would 'kill him'. This is always a tricky situation, and without going into the details I agreed to honour their request, but said I would be obliged to speak truthfully if he asked for details. It only took a few days before he sought an explanation. I sat down with him, his wife, their two children and his brother, and gently broke the news of his brain tumour. As he started to cry he was comforted by his two children. His wife, however, did not move and accused me of causing him unnecessary pain. To cut a long story short, he was discharged from hospital (at his request) and was readmitted approximately one month later. During this final admission, his brother thanked me for telling him the truth. In his final weeks, this man said good bye to those he loved and ensured his wife, who had previously been under the care of a psychiatrist, would continue to see him after his death. He died having completed all that he needed to do.

Generally, when asked a difficult or probing question, avoid giving an immediate answer. Instead, put the same question back to the one who posed it. You may say, "Tell me what you think?" This gives them the opportunity to unpack their thoughts and fears and for you to hear their pain. In many cases it is not an answer they want, but an opportunity to talk about their concerns. If they persist, however, move slowly and gently towards the truth. Most suspect the truth, and all you are doing is confirming their suspicions. There may be tears, but the news could also be greeted with silence or a stoical comment. If there are tears, do not feel it is because of what you said or how you said it. You have simply unlocked the floodgates and allowed your loved one to grieve openly. Be there with them, be present to their needs, but do not be afraid to grieve with them. Shedding a tear, even if their eyes are dry shows that you really care. Words are somewhat empty at this point and often go unheard, so a respectful silence and an appropriate level of physical contact are better ways of showing your compassion. At some point they will make the next move; allow them this, and be fully present to that moment. Truth telling may be one of the hardest things you have to do, but it is a most important step in midwifing the death of someone you love.

Chapter 6

Spiritual care

Chapter 6

Spiritual care

If I had to nominate one aspect of whole-person care that causes the most confusion it would be spiritual care. In this post-modern era, many believe that spiritual care (sometimes called pastoral care) is a devious way of introducing religion into the caring agenda. I hope to dispel this myth and show that spiritual care is central to whole-person care and fundamental to the healing process. Spiritual care deals with *why* and *what* questions, or as quantum physicists would say, the *hard* questions. For some, the inquiry may turn to religion and salvation, but for most it remains existential and personal in nature. In an effort to unpack this issue let us first explore the meaning of spirituality.

Spirituality

Again, there is a mistaken belief that spirituality, like spiritual care is all about a person's relationship with the sacred, the divine or some higher being, and has little to do with the material world. For this reason spirituality has been erroneously linked with religion or is considered so esoteric that many in this post-modern world see no need for it.

Spirituality is not necessarily esoteric or mysterious and is not linked *ipso facto* with religion; it deals with our deepest and innermost relationships with the unknown (Moody 1998). It addresses deep-seated questions like, "Who am I?", "What is the meaning and purpose of my life?", and "What will become of me?" A person's religious orientation may influence their response to these core questions, but no more than the values they live by, their culture, life experiences, and stage of life. What is important is that the absence of any religious belief does not negate this form of inquiry nor make the inquiry less relevant. The questions are pertinent to everyone, and while they may not rank high on the list of priorities for some, they inevitably come to the fore with increasing age, a personal crisis, and when confronted by the reality of impending death.

The early and middle adult years are generally orientated towards security and consolidation. The focus at this time of life is on the outer or material world. At some later stage, particularly with infirmity or in times of illness, the tendency is to focus more on one's inner life. Indian culture refers to this latter period as the 'years of wisdom'– the time a person prepares for death. The integral psychologist, Ken Wilber submits a similar analysis of life's unfolding when he says, "Spirit first throws itself outward to get lost in the [material] world and then begins the slow and tortuous return to Itself, finally to awaken as Itself" (1993: xviii). Put more simply, our formative and middle years are orientated towards the outer world. In later life the focus is on our inner world and the desire to discover who we really are. This path of discovery is spirituality in action, and is often referred to as the spiritual journey.

Why this inquiry is left to the eleventh hour is intriguing. According to Pierette Stukes, the majority of the population leads, what she calls, an outside-in existence where identity, meaning and purpose (the hard questions) are derived from our roles, our successes, our failures and what others think of us. When faced with a crisis or increasing age, the outside-in orientation loses its appeal and the search for a deeper meaning to life becomes more important. A shift away from this worldly (outside-in) orientation to an inside-out perspective occurs when, according to Stukes, we seek to know and express our true *self*. This is often the start of the spiritual journey and, metaphorically speaking, it involves shedding materialistic longings in favour of a reflective life.

This transition is not without pain. In the palliative care situation it involves a letting go of unrealistic hopes, and surrendering to the unknown. Such a quantum shift is only possible if family and healthcare workers respect and support the seeker as they struggle with their changing world. This is something an amicus may be called upon to facilitate.

The spiritual journey

The process of opening to and exploring our spirituality is, as previously mentioned, referred to as the spiritual journey. This journey may not be smooth. This is especially true for those facing death. There are always twists and turns, and countless bumps along the way. John O'Donohue suggests this journey is often a quarter inch long and several miles deep. Pain and soul-searching are intrinsic to it, but healing and peace are also possible, provided the suffering is confronted. Failure to explore the suffering can, however, lead to despair. In the words of Archbishop Desmond Tutu, "Unless you look the beast in the eye it returns to hold you hostage" (2009: 28). Those who receive bad news or experience a life-changing event are in urgent need of spiritual care. They need someone who can journey and be there with them as they confront their valley of darkness and the ultimate realisation that the life they once knew is forever changed.

Stephen Levine, in his book *Who Dies*, says the death of *self* is accompanied by much more pain than the death of the physical body. What he is emphasising is that spiritual, psychological and existential concerns are more common and more challenging for those who are dying than are their physical symptoms. What the dying want is help to overcome fear, particularly the fear of the unknown. The evidence, however, suggests that we fail them miserably. A recent patient satisfaction survey involving almost two million hospital inpatients in the USA found that emotional and spiritual care was lacking even though it was high on the patients' list of priorities (Koenig 2002 & 2008).

There are many reasons for this inconsistency. Often, the person's call for help goes unrecognised or is misinterpreted because of the metaphorical or symbolic language they are inclined to use. Other reasons include the low priority given to spiritual concerns, a fear of becoming emotionally involved, of getting out of one's depth, a perceived lack of time, or a belief that it is someone else's job. This is not meant to suggest that those in healthcare lack compassion, but rather they are often lost and unsure about how to care for those who are suffering. Their focus is generally on outcomes and making things better; an outside-in orientation.

Christine Bryden – a remarkably insightful woman living with dementia – says spirituality lies at the centre of our being, and is what identifies us to be truly human. She goes on to say, "We discover this spiritual essence whenever we pause long enough to look beyond cognition, through our clouded emotions into what lies within" (1998: 163). In this post-modern era there is, unfortunately little time given to reflection. For people in hospital, particularly those who have the most to gain, opportunities for reflection and introspection are few and far between.

Spiritual essence lies dormant until woken, often quite abruptly, by illness, a life crisis or by impending death. The amicus plays a vital role in helping their dying relative or friend awaken to it.

Spiritual care

Although I have used the words 'existential' and 'spiritual' interchangeably, the spiritual journey is as much psychological as it is existential. This link between the psyche and the spiritual is inseparable and the resolution of the hard questions is only possible if one deals with the emotions that underpin them – uncertainty, fear of impending death, the sense of dread or despair, paralysing anxiety, fear of the unknown, et cetera. Each person finds their own way through this maze and there is no set formula as to how this is done. Allowing a person to sit with their fear, their despair and their uncertainty is often the best course of action and is usually more valuable than trying to make sense of the incomprehensible.

Suffering is part of the spiritual journey and is an experience that has to be lived; it is not a problem that can be solved. From the amicus or midwife perspective, spiritual care is more about being and less about doing. It's listening and not rescuing.

To *be* with someone as they make this journey is hard work. The qualities required of such a person have been mentioned earlier, but now is a good time to refresh your memory. He or she is the friend (midwife), "... who can be silent with us in a moment of despair or confusion, who can stay with bereavement, who can tolerate not-knowing, not-curing, not-healing and face with us the reality of our powerlessness, that is the friend who cares" (Nouwen 1988). The difficulty in being this healing presence within a system which prioritises, expects, and rewards *doing* is immediately apparent. Fortunately there are people who are attuned to the needs of those who are dying and who do not seek to rescue or give advice. They are the ones who are prepared to listen. They correctly interpret the searching question, the subtle message or the pregnant pause to mean, "Can you hear my pain?" and willingly give of themselves and their time. That person may be a doctor, nurse, volunteer, pastoral care worker, cleaner or midwife. Whoever it may be, it is important to remember that they may, at some later time, need their own healing presence. Being with someone whose life is literally falling apart is hard work, and to suggest otherwise would be misleading.

While members of the healthcare team are in the front line of spiritual care, patients will often choose someone less involved to hear their pain. Unless prepared, this person may be overwhelmed. Being open and present to this possibility is, however, one of the hallmarks of an amicus.

The art of *being* is much more difficult for someone locked into a materialistic world as their focus is often on making things better – the *doing*. Anyone who seeks to midwife the death of another is well advised to pursue some form of reflective practice, and to look at their own fears and agendas around death; to take an inside-out look at their life and their work. When we are liberated from our fears, says Nelson Mandela, our presence automatically liberates others.

Chapter 7

Healing at the end of life

Chapter 7

Healing at the end of life

The spiritual or healing journey for someone who is dying may be long and tortuous. While this is true, it is also well known that healing can sometimes occur out of the blue. Why this happens is a mystery, but there is some evidence to suggest that the unconscious mind plays a part through the medium of dreams or deathbed experiences. In the context of death and dying, both can soothe a troubled mind and lead to a profound and unexpected healing. I touched on deathbed visions in Chapter 3 and would now like to take you on a short exploration of the world of dreams and the nature of unconsciousness.

Dreams

Dreams are the unconscious mind's attempt to resolve everyday issues. They have a message for us, but as the language and images are symbolic, the meaning can be confusing, and for those who remember their dream, it is often misinterpreted or ignored. If the dream is trying to convey something of importance, the unconscious will continue with its efforts, and the dream becomes recurrent until the conscious mind hears and comprehends what is being flagged. Dreams that are recurrent, nightmarish, explicit, or those that wake the dreamer are examples of the unconscious mind trying to alert us to something important. Not surprisingly, 'alerting' dreams are common amongst those who are dying, particularly if the person cannot or will not confront the reality of their situation (as was the case with Lou in Chapter 5).

Dreams around the time of death attempt to prepare the dying person for what is ahead. First and foremost they draw attention to the truth – that death is nigh. If this reality is denied, the dream imagery may become more explicit, leaving little to the imagination. One of my patients who could not accept he was dying had recurrent nightmares of being attacked from behind by a stranger wielding a dagger. The nightmares were so real and so frightening he feared sleep. The dream ultimately broke through the barrier his conscious mind had constructed, and for the first time he started to talk about his fear of death. At this point the nightmares ceased (Barbato 2010: 273).

We may not remember or recall our dreams, but dreams are a regular nightly occurrence. They arise from and are stored in a part of the brain which is inaccessible to the thinking, probing mind. This explains why we may have difficulty recalling them. This inaccessible part of our 'world' is called the *unconscious*. Not surprisingly then, dreams are our windows into the unknown, and were notoriously described by Freud as the royal road to the unconscious. Most dreams arise during rapid eye movement (REM) sleep, and seem to dissolve back to where they came immediately upon wakening. Although locked away and beyond reach of the waking mind (for most people), dreams continue to influence the way we feel over the ensuing days.

There is so much about dreams that we do not understand. What we do know is that they are more common and easier to recall with those who are dying. A possible reason for this could be the dearth of external rituals (in most Western cultures) surrounding death. Dugan says "In the absence of rituals, the human psyche seems to produce its own framework of significance [inner rituals] through symbolic images in dreams" (1989: 19-20). It could be said that dreams fill the gap that the medicalization of death has created, namely our neglect of rituals around the time of death. Dreams prepare the dying person for what lies ahead, and will do this irrespective of whether the dying person attends to them or not. According to one dream analyst,

> *"The unconscious will do its work whether or not the person attends to the dreams. This is true for people who cannot remember their dreams and even for those whose mentation is affected by the organic process of illness [e.g. dementia or delirium]"* (Muff 1996: 81).

Although their importance is all but ignored in the care of the dying, I have, in recent years made a habit of asking my patients about their dreams. Several reported troublesome or recurrent dreams and were grateful for the opportunity to talk about them. Simply by sharing, they came to understand what their dreams meant, and in all cases this set them on the path towards healing. Others found the opportunity to explore their dreams a pleasant diversion, and while there may not have been healing as such, there was some delight in talking about them. Asking about dreams, provided it is done at an appropriate time and in a caring manner can, at times, be a key element to midwifing death.

The significance of dreams at the end of life is, at last, being recognised and are now seen as profoundly meaningful and a source of great comfort for those who are dying. In a recent study, 87% of patients within one hospice were found to have a dream within weeks of their death (Kerr 2014). Most occurred during sleep, but a significant number carried into wakefulness and were interpreted by the dreamer as a vision rather than a dream. Interestingly, the majority of the dreams/visions were of deceased loved ones who, in turn, conveyed messages of both comfort and guidance to the dreamer. While confirming the healing potential of end-of-life dreams this study also raises the real possibility that deathbed visions may be the product of a vivid dream that has extended into waking consciousness. The debate concerning the nature and origin of deathbed visions will, no doubt, continue, but we should never lose sight of the fact that these dreams/visions, irrespective of their origin, are deeply meaningful and comforting to the dying patient, and that is what really matters.

Unconsciousness

Most of us are familiar with the words unconsciousness and coma, but few understand what they truly mean. In the medical literature, coma and unconsciousness are used interchangeably to describe a state where a person is unresponsive and seemingly unaware of what is happening to them. Unconsciousness can result from any number of causes including head injury, stroke, cardiac arrest, epilepsy, drug overdose, diabetic coma (from either excessively high or low blood sugar levels) and organ failure. Anaesthetic agents are commonly used to induce unconsciousness in those requiring surgery, and powerful sedation is occasionally employed in intensive care units to maintain comfort in ventilated or seriously ill patients. In the palliative care situation, the unconsciousness that commonly precedes death results from the underlying medical condition. Sedation can sometimes be a contributory factor, but pain relief medication such as morphine plays little or no part in its onset or progression.

The experience of unconsciousness has until recently been somewhat of a mystery. While many survive, few have been asked to describe what, if anything, they experienced during the unconscious period. Reports, however, are now appearing and what they tell us is surprising and instructive. While 25 percent have no memory for that time, the remaining 75 percent recalled things that were done to them, as well as things that were said to or about them. They also recalled dreams and were acutely aware of times when they felt fear and anxiety associated with their helpless, vulnerable and dependent state. On the positive side, many said how much they were helped by those who spoke to them, orientated them to what was happening, and forewarned them of any intervention such as a wash, an injection or a change of position (Lawrence).

Contrary to popular belief, most unconscious patients have a degree of awareness – particularly for touch and sound – which varies from moment to moment, and is particularly influenced by medical circumstances and the immediate environment. The ability to feel pain and touch, or to hear words and noise continues until the person recovers or, alternatively, until late in the dying process. How much an unconscious person understands, however, depends on what is being said and who says it. The more significant the person, and the more emotive the message, the more they remember. Evidence now indicates that those who are unconscious, including those close to death, gain considerable comfort from hearing the voice and feeling the touch of someone they love.

Indeed, there is now research to suggest that the ability to hear and appreciate touch is not only present, but may be more acute in those who are unconscious. A recent report in *Scientific American* has shown that blindfolding a person for as little as 90 minutes heightens the sense of touch by priming the visual as well as the sensory cortex to respond to it (Rosenblum 2013). Further research has also shown that hearing a familiar voice invokes neural activity involved in face recognition. This suggests that the unconscious person hears what is being said and may also visualise the face of the one speaking to them – providing, of course, that person was known to them beforehand. This cross sensory compensation is more prevalent than previously thought, but is greatly impaired with even moderate levels of background noise (Rosenblum 2013: 69). Not only does this confirm the importance of speaking to and making tactile contact with an unconscious loved one, it also reaffirms the need to create a healing environment and to eliminate unwanted background noise.

Bearing this in mind, I always suggest to those at the bedside that they speak to their dying and unconscious loved one as if he/she can hear – talk to them and not *about* them. Introduce themself (say their name) and greet them with a kiss or a touch. Orientate them to the time and the day, shower them with loving words and maintain some form of physical contact such as holding hands. Sit with them, and between periods of silence, read or sing to them, play music, brush their hair, massage their feet, and rub oil/cream into their skin. Tell them when you are about to leave and acknowledge this with a farewell touch or kiss. All this is comforting and healing not only for your dying relative but also for you.

An unconscious person can and does experience pain, so it is not uncommon for them to receive pain-relieving injections during this time. Family are often concerned that such treatment will render their relative more unconscious or hasten death. Pain medication, if given in appropriate doses to those who are unconscious, will not depress their level of awareness further, nor will it hasten death. Morphine and other analgesics simply relieve pain and ensure comfort. Pain rather than morphine is more likely to have a negative effect on the experience of dying.

While the state of unconsciousness that precedes death is similar to unconsciousness due to other causes, there are some important differences. The former is more akin to a deep sleep, and like sleep the dying person may open their eyes or wake fully (albeit temporarily). This may come out of the blue or may be related to a significant event, such as a long awaited relative arriving, or because of something that has been said. This awakening can also occur immediately before death and has all the hallmarks of a deathbed vision – the person opens their eyes and stares straight ahead as if they are looking at something or someone. After a brief time they simply lay back and breathe their last.

Death and the dying process is a mystery. The more a person midwifes death, the more they come to respect this mystery and the many gifts that are available for all that share the journey.

Epilogue

In the last 100 years, the care of the dying has moved from the home to a variety of healthcare facilities. While there are sound and pragmatic reasons for this change, it has effectively resulted in the loss of an art form that was once widely practiced. Family and friends who, in earlier times, midwifed the death of a loved one now run the real risk of becoming mere spectators as death becomes increasingly institutionalised and, in many cases, medicalised. Hopefully, this book has shown that midwifing death is possible irrespective of the circumstances, and is indeed desirable if the goal is to care for the *whole person.*

The four domains that have been identified as contributing to whole-person care are physical comfort, a healing environment, a healing presence and spiritual care. The art of midwifing death is to recognise the importance of the four domains and to ensure, as best as one can, that each is given due attention. Healing or peace in the face of death is more likely when the sick or dying person is free of pain, nursed in an environment that is precious to them, and is surrounded by family and friends of their choosing. The family's role in delivering physical comfort is significant, but their strength lies in the ability to attend to the other three domains – to be a trusted confidante who is present to the needs of their dying loved one.

> *"To have such a person at such a time is a great good fortune. To be that person, to have been such a person is a heavy and blessed experience. Once in each lifetime, we are meant to be a blessing [an amicus] to another"* (Lerner 1978: 133).

Let me conclude by telling you about Bill. I met Bill a matter of weeks before he died, but in this short time I got to know and respect him and his family. He exemplified for me the dignity and grace that goes with dying well, and how this can be facilitated by a family who is prepared to midwife the death of someone they love.

> *Bill had known for some time that death was imminent. Throughout this time he was supported and cared for [midwifed] by his family, his general practitioner and a team of community nurses. His decision to reject active treatment was accepted and understood, and he had time to continue his journey, safe in the knowledge he would not be abandoned. He grieved the loss of his wife, children, his friends, his dog, his work and his possessions. He prepared for his death, and when that time came he departed peacefully and without a struggle* (Barbato 1998).

I hope this book gives you the knowledge, skills and courage to be an amicus for a family member or friend as they confront serious illness and the possibility of death. The application of this knowledge is not, however, limited to the care of those who are dying. It can also be drawn on throughout life, particularly as you interact with people in need of a healing presence.

The eternity after death is simply the mirror image
of the eternity before birth

LUCRETIUS
1ST CENTURY GREEK PHILOSOPHER

Bibliography

Ariès, P. (1981). *The Hour of Our Death*. Middlesex: Penguin Books.

Barbato, M. Death is a journey to be undertaken. *MJA* 1998;168:296-297.

Barbato, M. (2009). *Reflections of a Setting Sun*. Self-published and available from www.caringforthedying.com.au

Barbato, M. (2010). *Caring for the Living and the Dying*. Self-published and available from www.caringforthedying.com.au

Barker, P. Working with the metaphor of life and death. *J Med Ethics: Medical Humanities* 2000;26:97-102.

Bell, H. R. (1998). *Men's Business, Women's Business – the spiritual role of gender in the world's oldest culture*. Rochester, Vermont: Inner Traditions.

Bryden, C. (1998). *Dancing with Dementia*. London: Jessica Kingsley Publishers.

Buckman, R. (1988). *I Don't Know What To Say*. Sydney: Sun Books.

Callahan, D. Pursuing a peaceful death. *Hastings Centre Report* (1993).23(4): 33-38.

Callahan, D. Death and the research imperative. *NEJM* 2000;342(9):654-656.

Campbell, J. (1995). *The Ars Moriendi – an examination, translation and collation of the manuscripts of the shorter Latin version*. http://www.ruor.uottawa.ca/fr/bitstream/handle/10393/10313/MM07840.PDF?sequence=1

Dugan, D. Symbolic expressions of dying patients: communication, not hallucination. *Nursing Forum* 1989;24(2):18-27.

Elliot, H. Moving beyond the medical model. *J of Holistic Healthcare* 2011;8:1-4.

Engel, G. The need for a new medical model: a challenge for biomedicine. *Science*, April 8, 1977.

Estle, K. Healing – the spiritual work of palliative care. *J of Palliative Medicine* 2013;16(1):106-7.

Fenwick, P & E (2008). *The Art of Dying*. NY: Continuum.

Grogono, J. A good death. *BMJ* 2000;320:1205.

Illich, I. *Death Undefeated*. http://ournature.org/~novembre/illich/1995_death.html.

Jones, G. (1998). *Magnanimous Despair*. Mt Nebo: Boombana Publications.

Kavanaugh, R. (1974). *Facing Death*. Baltimore: Penguin Books.

Kearney, M. (1996). *Mortally Wounded*. Dublin: Marino Books.

Kearney, M. (2000). *A Place of Healing*. Oxford: Oxford University Press.

Keeley, P. *Now and at the hour of our death: the Ars moriendi and modern dying*. *European Journal of Palliative Care* 2001;8(5):208-211.

Kellehear, A. (2000). *Death and Dying in Australia*. South Melbourne: Oxford University Press.

Kellehear, A. (2007). *A Social History of*

Dying. Port Melbourne: Cambridge University Press.

Kerr, C. et al. End-of-Life Dreams and Visions. *J of Palliative Medicine* 2014;17(3):296-303.

Koenig, H. (2002). *Spirituality in Patient Care.* Pennsylvania: Templeton Foundation Press.

Koenig, H. (2008). *Medicine, Religion and Health.* Pennsylvania: Templeton Foundation Press.

Kübler-Ross, E. (1970). *On Death and Dying.* London: Tavistock Publications Ltd.

Lamerton, R. (1980). *Care of the Dying.* Middlesex: Pelican Books.

Lawrence, M. (1997). *In a World of Their Own.* Connecticut: Bergin & Harvey.

Leget, C. Retrieving the ars moriendi tradition. *Medicine, Health Care and Philosophy* 2007;10:313-319.

Lerner, G. (1978). *A Death of One's Own.* New York: Simon and Schuster.

Levine, S. (1982). *Who Dies?* New York: Anchor Books

Lewis, M.J. (2007). *Medicine and Care of the Dying.* New York: Oxford University Press.

Livingston, G. (2000). *Only Spring.* Sydney: Hachette Australia.

Medawar, P. In T. Greenhalgh (Author). Intuition and evidence – uneasy bedfellows? *British Journal of General Practice* 2002;52:395-400.

Miller, J. (2001). *The Art of Being a Healing Presence.* Fort Wayne. Willowgreen Publishing.

Mitchell, S. (1991). *The Enlightened Mind.* New York: Harper Collins

Moody, H., Carroll, D. (1998). *The Five Stages of the Soul.* London: Rider.

Moody, R. (1975). *Life after Life.* Georgia: Bantam Books.

Moore, T. (1992). *Care of the Soul.* New York: HarperCollins.

Muff, J. (1996). From the wings of night. *Holistic nursing practice*; 10(4):69-87.

Nouwen, H. (1974). *Out of Solitude.* Notra Dame: Ave Maria Press.

Nouwen, H. (1988). *The Road to Daybreak: a spiritual journey.* New York: Doubleday.

Nouwen, H. (1995). *The Path of Waiting.* New York: Crossroad.

O'Donohue, J. (2004). *Anam Cara: A Book of Celtic Wisdom.* New York: Harper Perennial.

Remen, R.N. (1996). *Kitchen Table Wisdom.* Sydney: Pan Macmillan.

Rizzolatti., Fogassi. L., Gallese. V. Mirrors in the Mind. *Scientific American* (2006);295:54-61.

Rosenblum, L. A Confederacy of Senses. *Scientific American* 2013;308(1):67-69.

Sherman, B. (1999). *Dementia with Dignity.* Sydney: McGraw-Hill.

Stukes, P. Healing the postmodern soul. *Presence: an International Journal of Spiritual Direction* (2011);17(4):33-43.

Thomas, D. (1939). Do not go gentle into that good night. *The Poems of Dylan Thomas.* http://www.poetryfoundation.org/poem/175907

Tutu, D. (2009). *No Future Without Forgiveness.* New York: Image Doubleday.

Wilber, K. (1993). *The Spectrum of Consciousness.* Wheaton: Quest Books.

Wills-Brandon, C. (2000). *One Last Hug Before I Go.* Florida: Health Communications, Inc.

Midwifing Death Correspondence Course (MDCC)

This interactive correspondence course is designed to inform, empower and guide adults in the art of Midwifing Death. On completing the course, participants will have an enhanced understanding of the physical and psycho-spiritual needs of the sick and dying, and will be sufficiently skilled to become an amicus (friend and midwife) to any person living with a life-limiting or life-threatening illness.

Courses run over six months and will commence in February and July of each year. Participants submit six essays, attend a compulsory weekend workshop (a distance education option is available for those unable to attend the workshop; see later for details) and complete the required reading. The course facilitators are Michael Barbato, a palliative care physician, and Ann Barbato, a bereavement counsellor and yoga teacher. Both have many years of experience in their respective professional fields.

The course is divided into 14 modules as follows:

MODULE 1: Readings to get you started

Midwifing Death	MICHAEL BARBATO
The Art of Being a Healing Presence	JAMES MILLER
The Death of Ivan Ilyich	LEO TOLSTOY
On Death and Dying	ELISABETH KÜBLER-ROSS
Who Dies	STEPHEN LEVINE

These books embrace many of the course themes and contain information relevant to the essays in Modules 4-13. You can choose to read the books before attempting the essays or you may spread the reading over the entire course. The first two books are short and address the art of Midwifing Death directly. The remaining three are classics and 'must reads' for anyone interested in the subject of death and dying.

MODULE 2: Why become an amicus? (Compulsory essay)

An initial compulsory essay of up to 1000 words on the following topic: "Indicate your reasons for becoming an amicus (midwife to the sick and dying) and the challenges that may confront you in this role?" This essay is designed to orientate participants into the course, and help them gain insight into agendas, beliefs, and fears that could influence their role as an amicus. The module is to be completed and submitted at least two weeks before the weekend workshop (Module 3).

MODULE 3: Workshop

This compulsory weekend workshop will give course participants the opportunity to discuss and explore a range of challenging topics, including the role of an amicus in the 21st century. Experiential exercises will help promote a better understanding of beliefs and conditioning which may compromise the amicus role. This approach is in keeping with the wisdom espoused by Ken Wilber, who says, "The crucial ingredient is not the carer's bag with all the tricks, but the holder of that bag."

The workshop will take place in Kiama on a weekend to be nominated and will run from Saturday morning to Sunday lunch.

MODULE 4: Death in society (Compulsory essay)

One essay of up to 1000 words on one of the following three topics:

- Death from Eastern and Western perspectives
- The "D" word: community attitudes towards death and dying
- Death: a failure of treatment or a profound human experience?

Choose one essay from any three of the elective Modules 5-13

MODULE 5: End of life

5A: Suffering and the pain of dying

5B: Dying in hospital, and the medicalization of death

5C: Palliative care: philosophy and practice.

MODULE 6: Psycho-spiritual care

6A: Healing presence and healing environment

6B: The spiritual journey

6C: Healing and curing: the same or different?

MODULE 7: Communication

7A: Truth telling and the loving lie

7B: Responding to difficult questions

7C: The role of metaphor, intuition, music and art therapy.

MODULE 8: Death as a mystery

8A: Dreams

8B: Visions and nearing-death awareness

8C: Unconsciousness: is it a state of NO awareness?

MODULE 9: Special situations

9A: End-of-life care for those with dementia

9B: End-of-life care for the aged

9C: End-of-life care in hospital or intensive care

9D: End-of-life care for the young.

MODULE 10: Grief and loss

10A: The experience of grief

10B: The role of hope

10C: How children grieve.

MODULE 11: Practical matters

11A: Creating sacred spaces

11B: Advance Care Planning and Enduring Guardianship

11C: Funerals and rituals.

MODULE 12: Topical matters

12A: The rights of the dying

12B: Euthanasia and physician-assisted suicide

12C: Complimentary therapies and alternative practices.

MODULE 13: Any related topic of your choosing

MODULE 14:

What have I learnt about myself? (Compulsory essay)

This final essay has no word limit. The question to be addressed is, "What have I learnt about myself in this journey towards becoming an amicus to the sick and dying?" The issues you may wish to address include: What have I learnt about myself? Have my beliefs around death and dying altered? Is there anything I could attend to in my life in preparation for my own death?

You are invited to be open and creative with this assignment. Trust your intuition and feel free to use metaphor, drawings, poetry and imagery.

In preparation for this assignment it is recommended that you commence a journal from day one of the course and record significant insights and dreams along the way. The contents of the journal may provide valuable material for this final essay.

Course Fee and Recognition

A course fee of $170 covers all costs and includes a free copy of Michael's books *Caring for the Living and the Dying*, *Reflections of a Setting Sun* and *Midwifing Death*. A concessional rate of $100 is available for pensioners, the unemployed and those unable to meet the full course fee. Please note, course fees may increase over time in keeping with inflation.

Each person who satisfactorily completes the course will receive a certificate confirming their participation.

Distance Learning

Although the weekend workshop is an important part of the Midwifing Death Correspondence Course, distance can sometimes make attendance difficult. For this reason a modified version of the course will be offered at each intake to a limited number of people who are unable to participate in the weekend.

The distance learning course will include all Modules listed above except Module 3. In its place there will be three experiential exercises that can be done at home and a journal kept of significant events, dreams, emotional shifts, as well as thoughts that arise during over the six-month period. A summary of this journal will be submitted for review at the end of the course.

The exercises will address three core aspects of the weekend workshop

- beliefs and agendas
- listening
- suffering

Details of the exercises will be forwarded to students throughout the course. Upon completion of each exercise, the participant will be asked to reflect on the interaction and submit this in writing.

If necessary, a skype link can be arranged for the purpose of debriefing and discussion.

Those wishing to apply for the distant learning package should contact Michael by email before registering to ensure spots are still available.

For further information go to www.midwifingdeath.com.au or email Michael at Michael.barbato6@gmail.com

NOTES